Parenting Autistic Teens:

A Parent's Guide To Transitioning The Autistic Kid into an Independent Young Adult

Fiona Brown

Parenting Autistic Teens: A Parent's Guide To Transitioning The Autistic Kid into an Independent Young Adult

Copyright © [Fiona Brown] [2024]

Disclaimer

The information provided in this book is for general informational purposes only. While every effort has been made to ensure the accuracy and completeness of the contents, the author and publisher assume no responsibility for errors or omissions. The information presented in this book should not be considered as professional advice, and readers are encouraged to consult with appropriate professionals for specific guidance tailored to their individual needs.

About the Author

Fiona Brown is a passionate advocate for autism awareness and support, drawing from her own personal journey as a parent of an autistic child. With a deep commitment to making a difference in the lives of individuals and families affected by autism, Fiona shares her experiences, insights, and strategies to empower others on their own journeys.

Table of Contents

Introduction

Chapter 1: Understanding Autism Spectrum Disorder

Chapter 2: Navigating Adolescence: Challenges and Opportunities

Chapter 3: Preparing for Transition

Chapter 4: Employment and Vocational Skills

Chapter 5: Social Relationships and Community Engagement

Chapter 6: Emotional Well-being and Self-Advocacy

Chapter 7: Supporting the Whole Family

Chapter 8: Looking Toward the Future

Conclusion

Introduction

Greetings and welcome to the guide, "Parenting Autistic Teens: A Parent's Guide To Transitioning The Autistic Kid into an Independent Young Adult." If this book has found its way to you, it's likely you're a parent or guardian of a teen on the autism spectrum, and you're embarking on the complex adventure that is their teenage years, with the additional layer of ASD.

From personal experience, I'm intimately familiar with the special set of challenges, the moments of uncertainty, and the unexpected delights that accompany the task of guiding an autistic teenager into adulthood.

As you flip through these pages, please know that your experiences resonate with me. I share in the heavy cloak of concern you wear, the tender sorrow you feel watching your teen make their way in a world that can seem disorienting and unresponsive. I recognize the nights you lie awake fretting over what lies ahead for them, the fleeting doubts that haunt you, questioning whether your efforts are sufficient, whether you yourself are sufficient.

Raising an autistic teenager is a unique adventure, filled with its own highs and lows. You'll find yourself cheering for every victory, no matter how small, and sometimes grappling with moments of doubt and frustration. This path demands a blend of patience, tenacity, and unconditional love. More than anything, it's a path ripe with opportunities for personal and mutual growth, empowerment, and profound learning experiences for both you and your adolescent.

Parenting an autistic teenager isn't just an adventure—it's an emotional whirlwind, a maze of hurdles, and a powerful display of human resilience. It asks for your all—your time, your patience, your grit—and in return, it blesses you with instances of indescribable joy and deep connection.

My Own Story: The Reason Behind the Book

Before we dive deep into the subject, let me share a bit of my own story and what drove me to pen this book.

Like many of you, I began this journey with a mix of apprehension and uncertainty. I wondered if I had what it takes—the knowledge, the skills, the resources—to support my autistic teenager in blossoming. I relentlessly sought out answers, digging through every resource I could find for some guidance and peace of mind.

I didn't write this book claiming to be an expert. Rather, I wrote it as someone who's right there with you on this rocky road, someone who's had their fair share of falls but keeps pressing on. I wrote it because I've been in your position, enduring the sharp glances of strangers and the silent tears of overwhelm. My goal in writing is straightforward: to provide you with the support, advice, and comfort you need as you and your autistic teenager navigate the journey from adolescence into adulthood. Within these pages lies a treasure trove of hands-on advice, relatable stories, and insights that come from a place of empathy.

But my motivation also came from the incredible highs—the sheer happiness when my teenager made their first real friend, the overwhelming pride at witnessing them overcome a challenge we once thought impossible. I wrote this book because I have faith in the enduring strength of the human spirit and the transformative power of love, even on the toughest days.

Through a process of trial and error, I've picked up essential lessons on raising an autistic teenager—lessons I'm eager to pass on to others walking this path. I've discovered that while the journey can be demanding, it's equally fulfilling. I've realized that with the right mix of support, resources, and mindset, our autistic teenagers can accomplish amazing feats.

Here, you won't stumble upon lofty theories or generic fixes. Instead, you'll encounter the genuine, unvarnished reality of parenting an autistic teenager—the ups and downs, the triumphs and obstacles, the moments of despair and hope that shape our experiences. You'll find actionable advice forged from real-life experience, stories that resonate with your own, and a deep sense of empathy—a reminder that you're never alone.

As we set out on this path together, rest assured that I'm here for you, ready to lend support and advice whenever you're in need. Your struggles are recognized, your pain is shared, and your journey is truly worth celebrating. In these pages, you'll find not just a guide, but a friend—someone who gets it, who cares, and who believes in the potential of you and your teenager.

Chapter 1: Understanding Autism Spectrum Disorder

What is Autism Spectrum Disorder (ASD)?

As a parent with a teenage child on the autism spectrum, it's crucial to get to grips with the basics of Autism Spectrum Disorder (ASD). Autism is a multifaceted neurodevelopmental disorder that influences the way an individual experiences the world, interacts with people, and processes information. Although the precise origins of autism are still a mystery, it's believed that a mix of genetic and environmental elements contributes to its emergence.

Autism typically involves distinct social communication and interaction styles, as well as limited and repetitive behavior patterns, interests, or activities. These traits can vary widely, from mild to profound, and can change over time. A key sign of autism is the challenge with social communication, which might include difficulty in picking up social cues such as gestures, facial expressions, and the tone of voice. For instance, your teen might find it hard to look someone in the eye while talking or to grasp indirect language like sarcasm or idioms.

Moreover, teens with autism might find starting and maintaining social interactions tough, which can lead to a sense of isolation or loneliness. Your teen may prefer to be alone or have a hard time making friends due to a misunderstanding of social norms and expectations.

Sensory sensitivities are also prevalent in those with autism. Many experience either intense or reduced responses to sensory input like sound, light, texture, or smell. This could mean that your teen feels stressed in busy places, is irritated by certain types of clothing, or seeks out particular sensory experiences for comfort.

Being aware of your teen's sensory preferences is key to crafting a supportive environment that reduces sensory overload and enhances their comfort and well-being.

Individuals with autism often show restricted and repetitive behavior, interests, or activities. These can manifest in various ways, such as repetitive motions (like hand-flapping or rocking), a strong need for set routines, or a deep interest in specific topics.

Although these behaviors might be comforting or serve as coping mechanisms for your teen, they can also pose challenges in everyday life. For example, a strict need for routine might make it tough to handle changes in schedule, while a narrow range of interests could restrict your teen's involvement in different activities.

It's essential to understand that autism doesn't look the same in everyone. Every person with autism is unique, with their individual strengths, challenges, and personality. As a parent, adopting the concept of neurodiversity – the view that neurological differences are to be acknowledged and valued – can aid you in helping your teen to accept their identity and find their niche in the world.

By getting to know the main features of autism spectrum disorder and how they appear in your teen, you're in a better position to meet their needs and encourage their personal growth and development. In the next sections, we'll delve into effective ways to handle the hurdles of autism while acknowledging and nurturing the strengths and possibilities of your autistic teen.

Getting a handle on the distinct traits of autism is key to supporting your child in the best way possible. Autism isn't uniform; it's a spectrum, meaning its impact varies from person to person. We'll look into the wide array of characteristics often observed in autistic individuals, using real-life scenarios and actionable advice.

The Unique Characteristics of Autism

Autism Spectrum Disorder (ASD) covers a wide variety of behaviors, competencies, and challenges. Your child's autism experience is as individual as they are, complete with their own set of strengths and areas for growth. Some autistic individuals might need significant support in their daily activities, while others may have remarkable talents and skills. Many are somewhere in the middle.

For example, consider Alex, a teenager on the spectrum who has a knack for mathematics but finds socializing tricky. Although making friends and reading social signals are challenging for him, his numerical abilities are impressive. Recognizing this range of skills can help parents embrace their child's distinct talents and hurdles.

One of the defining aspects of autism is hurdle with social communication. Your child might struggle to interpret non-verbal signals such as facial expressions and body language.

Starting and keeping up with conversations can be hard, and autistic individuals might not use many gestures or facial expressions to show how they feel.

Here's a Tip: *Get your teen to work on their social skills by trying out role-play or using social stories.*

Simplify tricky social stuff into easier bits, and give them a high-five for every win!

A lot of folks on the autism spectrum process senses differently, which can mean being super sensitive to stuff like sounds, textures, or lights. Some sensations can be too much and stressful, while others are just what they need to feel good.

For Example: *The noise from a vacuum cleaner is just too much for Alex. To make it better, his family either uses noise-blocking headphones or they vacuum when he's out.*

Autistic kids often like doing the same things over and over, like flapping their hands or sticking to a strict routine. They can also get really into certain subjects.

Restricted and repetitive behaviors are common in autism. Your child may engage in repetitive movements like hand-flapping or have rigid routines and rituals. They might develop intense interests in specific topics, devoting countless hours to learning everything about them.

These repeat behaviors mean something, like comfort or feeling safe. Don't just say no to them; instead, find ways to fit them in while gently nudging your child to try new stuff.

Understanding autism means getting the idea of neurodiversity – that brain differences are cool and should be celebrated. Cheer on your child's special talents and ways of seeing the world, and help them feel good about themselves.

For Example: Mark loves trains, so his folks take him to train museums and rides, which makes him happy and teaches him things like patience and focusing on details.

Autism comes with challenges, sure, but also with awesome strengths and interests. Find out what makes your child light up, whether it's a hobby, a favorite topic, or a special skill. Cheer them on to go after what they love and to try new things.

Keep in mind that what your child is into might change, and that's totally fine. Push them to be curious and to step out of their comfort zone. By doing this, you're helping them grow and see the world in new ways.

As you go through the adventure of raising an autistic child, keep an open mind and be ready to learn and grow with them. Celebrate their unique autism, back them up when things get tough, and stand up for what they need with love and guts. Together, we can build a world that gets neurodiversity and appreciates the many sides of autism.

Common Challenges Faced by Autistic Teens

If you've got an autistic teen, you know this time can be full of special challenges. Let's talk about what these might be and how you can be there for your teen with a lot of heart and smarts.

1. **Social Challenges:**

Socializing can be super confusing and tiring for autistic teens. Figuring out social hints, starting chats, or getting what people mean without words can be tough. This can make them feel alone, upset, and stressed out around others.

For Example: Sarah doesn't get the jokes and sarcasm from her classmates, leaving her feeling out of the loop at lunchtime. Her parents help her practice social skills with role-playing and give her scripts for common situations.

Here's a Tip: Set up chances for your teen to hang out where they feel comfy and have support. Maybe a small get-together with close pals or joining a group that works on social skills with a pro.

2. Getting Organized:

Skills like keeping things in order, managing time, and figuring out what to do first can be real hurdles for autistic teens. They might have a hard time remembering homework, sticking to routines, or switching from one thing to another.

For Example: Alex keeps forgetting his homework because organizing and time management are tricky for him. His parents help by making a visual schedule and using timers to keep him on track.

Here's a Tip: *Break tasks into smaller steps and use tools like checklists and calendars to help your teen stay sorted. Set up regular routines to give their day some predictability.*

3. Sensory Overload:

A lot of autistic teens are really sensitive to things around them, which can make normal places feel too intense and stressful. Loud noises, bright lights, or busy spots can lead to meltdowns.

For Example: *Mark gets overwhelmed in places like malls. His parents always have noise-canceling headphones and a fidget toy ready, so he's got ways to deal with too much sensory input.*

Here's a Tip: *Make home and other spaces more sensory-friendly by cutting down on stuff that bugs your teen. Give them things like headphones, shades, or stress balls to help them manage their senses.*

4. Growing Up:

As autistic teens get closer to being adults, they face the big job of learning to be independent. Things like taking care of themselves, cooking, or getting around by themselves can be hard. They might need help with money, finding work, or using community help.

For Example: The thought of growing up scares Alex. He's not sure about handling money or getting a job. His parents work with him on life skills like budgeting, cooking, and writing a resume to get ready for more independence.

Here's a Tip: Start teaching independence skills early and introduce new tasks slowly. Help them learn step-by-step and be there to guide them as they tackle grown-up challenges.

5. Mental Health and Well-being:

Autistic teens can be more likely to have mental health issues like anxiety or depression. They might not be great at sharing their feelings or asking for help, which can delay getting the right support. Plus, they might face unfair treatment when they try to get help.

For Example: Emily often feels anxious and overwhelmed because of sensory overload. Her parents make sure her mental health is a priority by teaching her ways to calm down, like mindfulness, and getting her therapy.

Here's a Tip: Talk openly about mental health and feelings with your teen, so they know it's okay to share and ask for help. Encourage them to do things that help them feel good, like working out, chilling out, or being creative.

6. Bullying and Social Exclusion:

Autistic teens can be picked on or left out because they communicate and act differently. This can make them feel lonely, hurt their self-esteem, and cause mental health problems.

For Example: Jake gets bullied at school because he has a hard time with social stuff and is sensitive to things around him. His parents stand up for him by talking to the school and giving him support and tools to handle the tough emotions.

Here's a Tip: *Teach your teen how to spot and deal with bullying, like learning to stand up for themselves and reaching out to adults they trust. Help them find friends who get them and like them just as they are.*

Parenting an autistic teen has its ups and downs, but with patience, love, and hard work, you can help your kid get through the teen years feeling strong and ready for what's next. By focusing on what they're good at, helping them through the rough spots, and speaking up for what they need, you're setting them up to rock their adult life. In the next parts of this guide, we'll dive into more ways and resources to back up your autistic teen as they step into the grown-up world.

Wrapping up Chapter 1, we've seen that helping an autistic teen through their journey is a mix of challenges and wins. We've shared tips and stories to help your teen grow and feel good about themselves. From making friends in the right places, to getting organized, to making sure their voice is heard at school, every step is about giving your child the power to shine.

As we've been making our way through these hurdles, we've looked into all sorts of handy tactics and actual stories designed to boost your teenager's growth and happiness. Whether we're talking about helping them make friends in places where they feel at ease, slicing up jobs into bits they can easily tackle, or standing up for what they need at school, every tactic is about giving your kid the tools to shine.

The leap from being a teen to becoming an adult is huge, packed with changes and discoveries for both you and your young one. It's the perfect moment to cheer on their special talents and to be there for them as they face any bumps in the road with kindness, patience, and solid support. By laying down a base of love, acceptance, and advice, you're setting your autistic teenager up to handle this time of change with a bunch of confidence.

Keep in mind, you're not flying solo on this trip. The experiences and tactics we've shared in this guide are proof that there's a whole community of folks out there facing similar things. Together, we're equipping our autistic teenagers with the right stuff to flourish as they step into the grown-up world.

In the next chapters, we're going to dive into specific growth and independence areas, offering even more in-depth advice and resources to help you and your autistic teenager on this path. Let's tackle the tough spots and throw a party for every win, no matter the size, as we guide our teens toward a future that's bright and full of promise.

Chapter 2: Navigating Adolescence - Challenges and Opportunities

The Adolescent Experience: A Neurodiverse Perspective

Making your way through the teenage years is a wild ride filled with all sorts of feelings, social scenes, and personal growth. For those on the autism spectrum, these years have their own set of twists and turns that mix with the usual teen stuff. In this part, we're going to look closer at what it's like to be a teen with a unique perspective, sharing insights, stories from real life, and smart moves to help both parents and teenagers steer through this key time.

Neurodiversity is about understanding that brain differences, like autism, ADHD, and dyslexia, are just part of the variety of human life. It's super important to help your teen see that their unique brain wiring isn't a mistake or a limit; it's just part of what makes them them. Shine a light on the cool things that come with their unique brain, like being super focused on details, being creative, or being a whiz at solving problems.

Teen years come with a lot of social puzzles, from making friends to getting the hang of unwritten social rules. Autistic teens might find this extra tricky because of challenges with chatting and reading body language. Help them by teaching social skills in a clear way, breaking down complex social stuff into steps they can manage. Using role-play and real-life situations can be a game-changer for practicing social skills in a place that's got their back. Push them to find their tribe where they're celebrated for being themselves, building a sense of belonging and connection.

This time in life is also when emotions run high and hormones are all over the place, so learning to keep emotions in check is super important for teens. Autistic teens might have an even tougher time with their feelings because of things like being extra sensitive to their surroundings and finding it hard to put their feelings into words. Teach them solid ways to handle stress, nerves, and feeling overwhelmed, like deep breathing, being mindful, and using sensory stuff that helps them feel calm. Make a space where they can talk about their feelings freely and without being judged, making sure their emotions are taken seriously and giving them support and advice when they need it.

Real-Life Example:

When Alex hit his teen years, he started bumping into more social hurdles at school. We picked out specific social skills he wanted to get better at, like starting chats and figuring out what people's faces were saying. We practiced these skills with role-play and real-life situations, and slowly but surely, he got more confident and skilled in social settings. Over time, Alex got the hang of social cues and came up with his own ways to handle social stuff with more ease and confidence.

By getting what it's like to be a teen with a different view and offering the right kind of help and advice, parents can give their autistic teens the power to go through these big changes with toughness, confidence, and a strong sense of self-worth. With patience, understanding, and getting ahead of problems, parents and teens can team up to tackle challenges and grab hold of the chances for growth and finding out who they are that come with being a teen.

By getting what it's like to be a teen with a different view and offering the right kind of help and advice, parents can give their autistic teens the power to go through these big changes with toughness, confidence, and a strong sense of self-worth. With patience, understanding, and getting ahead of problems, parents and teens can team up to tackle challenges and grab hold of the chances for growth and finding out who they are that come with being a teen.

Opportunities for Growth and Development

As your autistic teen wanders through their teen years, it's key to spot all the chances they have to grow, learn, and become their best selves. In this chapter, we're going to talk about how to make the most of these chances to help your teen find out what they're good at, chase what they love, and lay the foundation for a life they're excited about.

Getting your teen to dive into what they're into is crucial for giving them a sense of purpose and happiness. Whether they're into drawing, music, science, or sports, give them chances to get their hands dirty and get better at what lights them up. Check out workshops, classes, or local events that are all about what they're into, letting them sink into activities that make them happy and proud.

Building Resilience:

Teen years are sure to throw some curveballs, but they're also a chance for your teen to get tougher and learn to adapt. Teach them how to deal with letdowns, roll with changes, and come back from tough times. Push a mindset that's all about growing by making sure they know that messing up is just part of learning and a chance to get even better. Help them see the upsides of slip-ups, focusing on what they've learned instead of getting stuck on what didn't go right.

Real-Life Tip:

When Alex didn't make the basketball team and was feeling down, we talked about how important it is to keep going and not give up. We looked for other ways he could stay active and into sports, and that's when we found out he was a natural at swimming. Through this, Alex learned the value of not giving up and the importance of jumping on new chances, which led him to totally rock a sport he ended up loving.

Help your teen set goals that are doable and line up with what they're good at, what they like, and what matters to them. Break big goals into smaller steps, and make a big deal out of every step they nail. This doesn't just build confidence; it also gives them a sense of control and power. Push your teen to think about what they really care about, helping them pick goals that mean something to them.

By seeing and grabbing the unique chances for getting better and growing that come with being a teen, you can help your autistic teen go through this big time of change with toughness, self-belief, and a clear sense of what they want. With understanding, empathy, and being there for them, you can help them play to their strengths, chase what they love, and start on a path of finding out who they are and getting better every day.

Chapter 3: Preparing for Transition

Shifting from the teenage years into adult life marks a profound change for anyone, yet for those on the autism spectrum, it's a process that demands careful thought and assistance. In this section of thebook, we're going to look at why it's crucial to start planning early. We'll examine various paths for schooling, work, and self-reliance. Through sharing stories from real life and offering hands-on guidance, we're here to help you provide the support your teen needs during this pivotal time.

The Importance of Early Planning for Transition

The leap into adulthood is thrilling but can also be a bit overwhelming, especially if you're the parent of an autistic teenager like my own son, Alex. The secret to a smooth transition is to begin planning well in advance. It's all about preparing the ground for Alex to enter adulthood with confidence, equipped with the necessary abilities, ambitions, and a network of support to flourish.

Why Start Early?

Kicking off the transition planning early, even as early as middle school, gives you plenty of time to explore passions, build skills, and start introducing the idea of independence at a comfortable pace. This forward-looking strategy allows for tweaks to be made based on your teen'schanging interests and capabilities, keeping his transition plan fresh and in line with what he wants for his future.

Real-Life Example: Planning with Alex

For Alex, we started mapping out his journey to adulthood in middle school. We made sure he had u say in the process by setting up regular family chats to talk about his future. These weren't stiff, formal meetings, but relaxed discussions over dinner where Alex could feel at ease and valued. We covered his hopes, his favorite activities, and his vision for his future, touching on further education, career possibilities, and the kind of help he might need to live on his own.

One of Alex's early ambitions was to delve into graphic design, an area where he had shown considerable interest. Identifying this early on allowed us to seek out high school classes and after-school programs that would nurture his enthusiasm and talents.

Practical Tips for Effective Transition Planning

- **Create a Comprehensive Transition Plan:** Begin with a comprehensive plan that showcases your teen's strong points, hobbies, needs, and objectives. This plan is more than just a piece of paper; it's a guide to the future. It should outline long-term dreams, like career aspirations, and short-term targets, such as mastering public transport on their own.

- **Involve a Team:** The best transition plans come from teamwork. This team should include your teen, family, teachers, therapists, and other key figures in his life. Their combined insights ensure a well-rounded approach to planning, addressing different facets of your child's growth and future requirements.

- **Set Clear, Achievable Goals:** Goals should be specific, measurable, attainable, relevant, and time-bound (SMART). For Alex, an initial goal could be to finish a beginner's course in graphic design, either online or through a local program. These goals need clear deadlines and steps for success, making progress feel real and motivating.

- **Build Skills Gradually:** Understand that gaining independence and moving into adulthood doesn't happen overnight. Break down skills into smaller, more manageable tasks. For instance, if your teen's aim is to live on his own, start with simpler tasks like organizing his schedule or making basic meals, and then gradually move on to more complex life skills.

- **Review and Adapt:** The transition plan should be dynamic, regularly reviewed, and updated to reflect your child's changing needs, accomplishments, and dreams. Celebrate the goals he achieves and use any setbacks as chances to learn and refine the plan as necessary.

By getting an early start and focusing on a thorough, inclusive method to transition planning, we can help our teens to build a future that aligns with their strengths and dreams. It's all about empowering them to make informed choices, gain independence, and ultimately enjoy a satisfying adult life.

Guiding Your Teen Through Education, Work, and Independence

The journey to adulthood for teens is filled with chances for personal growth and discovery. This chapter zeroes in on steering your teen through education, employment, and self-reliance, with a focus on supportive tactics that fit their unique needs and goals.

Education: Nurturing Academic and Personal Growth

Moving on to higher education is a big step into a new realm of knowledge and self-exploration. It's essential to find a setting where your teen feels supported and can excel both in their studies and socially.

Supportive Strategies:

Identify Supportive Programs: Find colleges with specialized services for autistic students, which might include academic help, tutoring, social groups, and counseling. These resources can make a huge difference in your teen's college life.

Prepare for New Routines: Help your teen get used to the idea of college. Talk about what to expect, visit campuses in advance, and practice new daily routines to make the transition smoother.

Embrace Accommodations: Encourage your teen to make use of all available accommodations. Understanding and using these resources is key to managing workload and stress.

Employment: Fostering a Fulfilling Career Path

Securing a meaningful job means matching your teen's passions and abilities with the right opportunities. It's about creating a path that recognizes their unique skills and allows for professional growth.

Supportive Strategies:

Skill Development: Encourage your teen to take part in vocational training or internships in areas they're interested in. These experiences are priceless for picking up practical skills and getting a feel for the working world.

Seek Autism-Friendly Opportunities: There are many organizations and programs out there aimed at helping people on the autism spectrum. These can provide a more accommodating and understanding workplace for your teen.

Build a Support Network: Assist your teen in finding mentors and peers who can offer advice, support, and encouragement. This network can be vital for navigating the working world.

Independence: Empowering Self-Sufficiency and Confidence

Achieving independence means mastering key life skills and making informed choices about where to live in the future. It's about giving your teen the power to lead a life they decide for themselves.

Supportive Strategies:

Life Skills Development: Slowly introduce your teen to different life skills, like managing money, cooking, and personal care. Use straightforward instructions and visual aids to make learning easier.

Discuss Living Arrangements: Have open discussions about various living situations, taking into account your teen's preferences and needs for support. This could mean looking into communities with support or ways to live independently.

Promote Decision-Making: Get your teen involved in making decisions that affect their life, from everyday choices to big life changes. This helps build a sense of independence and confidence.

By using these strategies, you're not just preparing for your teen's move to adulthood; you're giving them the tools and confidence they need for the future. Every step is a building block toward a rewarding adult life, full of growth, self-discovery, and autonomy. The path might have its challenges, but with the right support and prep, your teen can step forward with assurance, ready to grab the opportunities that await.

Chapter 4: Employment and Vocational Skills

Exploring Career Paths

Guiding your child through career exploration is a transformative process of self-discovery, helping them to reveal their interests, talents, and goals. This section offers helpful approaches to assist them in examining a variety of career possibilities and pinpointing those that resonate with their abilities and enthusiasms.

Supportive Strategies:

Self-Exploration: Motivate your child to partake in introspective activities to pinpoint their passions, principles, and strong suits. This might include writing in a journal, taking personality tests, or chatting about which pursuits make them feel most alive. Understanding themselves better equips them to focus on career paths that match their individuality.

Research and Information Gathering: Aid your child in digging into diverse career fields to understand job roles, necessary skills, and opportunities for advancement. Use online tools like career portals, sector analyses, and professional group websites to learn about different fields and roles. Encourage a deep dive into their interest areas, examining various positions and career progressions.

Volunteering and Internships: Help your ward to get practical exposure through volunteer work, internships, or part-time gigs in areas they're curious about. Volunteering can introduce them to different sectors and job functions, while internships offer valuable experience and networking chances, aiding in making educated career decisions.

By fostering a spirit of self-discovery, supporting thorough research, and enabling real-world experiences, you're equipping them with the confidence and tools required for career exploration. Celebrate every step they take and cheer them on to pursue their passions and dreams as they consider their career options.

Developing Job Skills and Securing Work

Helping your child develop job skills and find suitable work is key to their successful entry into the workforce. This section focuses on ways to build relevant skills and find job opportunities that suit their strengths and interests.

Supportive Strategies:

Skill Development: Identify and focus on job skills that are pertinent to your child's career aspirations. Offer them chances to enhance their abilities through vocational training, workshops, online classes, and practical experiences.

Job Readiness Training: Provide them with crucial job readiness skills, like crafting resumes, preparing for interviews, honing communication abilities, and understanding workplace decorum. Practice interviews and role-play can bolster their confidence and skill set in these areas.

Networking and Job Search Strategies: Support your child in establishing professional connections and seeking out job opportunities. Encourage them to attend job expos, network meets, and industry gatherings. Use online job platforms, networking websites, and advice from mentors to help in their search.

Through career exploration and skill development, they're embarking on a path toward meaningful work and job satisfaction. With your backing, they can tackle the job market's complexities and chase opportunities that align with their passions and capabilities. Each step forward is a valuable learning experience that contributes to their growth and success in the working world.

Chapter 5: Social Relationships and Community Engagement

Navigating Social Relationships

Mastering social relationships is crucial for your child's development. This section shares tactics to help kids like Alex forge meaningful bonds while managing the intricacies of social interactions.

Supportive Strategies:

Social Skills Development: Give them plenty of chances to enhance their social abilities. Encourage your child to start conversations, make eye contact, and listen actively. Role-playing and social groups are great for building their social confidence.

Building Friendships: Create opportunities for them to meet peers with similar interests and values. Promote their involvement in activities and groups where they can find friends. Encourage shared experiences and open communication to foster real friendships.

Understanding Boundaries: Teach your teen about personal space and respecting others' limits. Help them recognize when someone feels uncomfortable and respond with empathy. Have open talks about boundaries and model good communication in your interactions with them.

Conflict Resolution Skills: Arm your teen with the skills to handle conflicts positively. Teach them to express themselves clearly, listen to others, and work towards solutions. Encourage approaching disagreements with empathy and a readiness to compromise.

Seeking Support: Encourage your teen to reach out to trusted people when facing social challenges. Offer a supportive space for them to talk about their experiences and seek advice.

With these strategies, your child can confidently navigate social relationships and build rewarding connections. With patience and support, they can develop relationships that enhance their life and contribute to their happiness.

Community Engagement: Connecting with Others

Getting involved in the community can greatly benefit your teen, offering personal growth and a chance to contribute. This section explores ways to actively participate in community life, fostering connections and meaningful involvement.

Supportive Strategies:

Volunteer Opportunities: Encourage your child to seek out volunteer work that aligns with their interests. Volunteering can provide a sense of purpose and valuable experiences while helping others.

Community Events and Clubs: Help your teen get involved in community events, clubs, and organizations that spark their interest. From sports teams to cultural festivals, there are many ways to connect and grow within the community.

Support Groups and Advocacy: Connecting them with support groups and advocacy organizations focused on topics relevant to him, such as autism awareness and acceptance, fosters a sense of belonging and empowerment. These groups provide a platform for sharing experiences, receiving support, and advocating for important causes.

By embracing these supportive strategies and actively engaging with the community, your teen can cultivate a sense of belonging, connection, and purpose in their life.

Chapter 6: Emotional Well-being and Self-Advocacy

Based on personal experiences, this section digs into the critical need to enhance emotional well-being and empower teens with autism to stand up for themselves.

Promoting Emotional Well-being

Supporting the emotional well-being of autistic teens is necessary for their holistic development and quality of life. Here's how you can promote emotional well-being:

Emotional Awareness: Help your child to get to know their own emotions. Use tools like picture cards, social narratives, or feelings charts to assist them in recognizing and sharing their emotions. This kind of emotional insight gives your child the skills to handle their feelings more effectively.

Coping Mechanisms: Teach your child ways to cope with stress and anxiety. This might include deep breathing, sensory items, or calming activities like listening to music or being outdoors. Discovering what suits your child best equips them with essential strategies for emotional regulation.

Social Support: Create a nurturing space where your teen can freely share their emotions and seek help when necessary. Promote open dialogue at home and encourage your child to form close bonds with peers and trusted adults. Having a network to rely on can greatly benefit your child's emotional health.

The Importance of Self-Advocacy

Self-advocacy is all about enabling those with autism to voice their needs and rights confidently. Here's how to foster these skills in your child:

Know Your Child's Rights: Learn and teach your child about their rights as a person with autism. Get to know legislation like the Individuals with Disabilities Education Act (IDEA) or the Americans with Disabilities Act (ADA). Knowing these rights strengthens your child's ability to stand up for themselves in different environments.

Effective Communication: Help your teen develop strong communication skills to express their needs and choices with assurance. Use role-play to practice speaking up in various scenarios, like asking for help at school or stating their preferences in social settings.

Problem-Solving Skills: Give your teen the tools to tackle problems and advocate for themselves effectively. Encourage them to think of solutions, seek help when necessary, and take active steps to address challenges. Cultivating a problem-solving mindset instills independence and resilience in your child.

By focusing on your child's emotional health and self-advocacy skills, you help them face life's hurdles with confidence and strength. Each step you take in supporting your child's emotional and self-advocacy journey shows your deep commitment as a caregiver.

Chapter 7: Supporting the Whole Family

Caring for a child with autism deeply affects the whole family. This section examines the various ways in which autism affects the family dynamic and provide strategies for supporting the well-being and harmony of the entire family unit.

The Impact on the Family:

Autism brings a mix of joys and challenges for a family. From the diagnosis to daily life and seeking support, every part of family life can be touched by the unique needs of the child with autism. Siblings might feel a range of emotions, from affection to frustration, as they interact with their autistic brother or sister. Parents often juggle the demands of caregiving with their other responsibilities.

Strategies for Family Support and Harmony:

- ***Open Communication:*** Encourage everyone in the family to share their thoughts and feelings openly. Set aside time for family discussions to talk about hurdles, celebrate successes, and brainstorm solutions.

- ***Education and Understanding:*** Educate family members about autism and its impact on behavior, communication, and social interaction. Help siblings understand their autistic sibling's unique needs and strengths, fostering empathy and acceptance. Provide age-appropriate resources and books that explain autism in a way that siblings can understand.

- ***Emotional Support:*** Provide emotional support for each family member, recognizing their individual challenges. Let siblings express their feelings and validate their experiences.

Encourage parents to seek support from each other, friends, or professionals.

- ***Division of Responsibilities:*** Share caregiving tasks fairly among family members. Consider each person's abilities and limits, and assign duties accordingly. Encourage collaboration and teamwork in managing daily routines and supporting the autistic child's development and well-being.

- ***Self-Care:*** Make self-care a priority for everyone, including parents, siblings, and extended family. Encourage breaks and activities that bring happiness and rest. Recognize that self-care is key to everyone's physical and emotional health.

- ***Celebrate Achievements:*** Acknowledge each family member's achievements, including the autistic child. Find ways to celebrate progress and value each person's strengths. Build a positive, resilient family culture, focusing on abilities rather than challenges.

By using these strategies, families can create a supportive atmosphere that promotes the well-being of each member, including the child with autism. Through open communication, learning, support, and self-care, families can face autism's challenges together and thrive.

Chapter 8: Looking Toward the Future

For parents of autistic individuals, looking to the future can be filled with hope and concern. This section looks at what comes after the teen years and offers resources for ongoing support and development.

Envisioning the Future: Beyond Adolescence

Navigating the transition from adolescence to adulthood is a pivotal moment for autistic individuals and their families. Here's how you can prepare for the journey ahead:

- *Identifying Strengths and Interests:* Spend time recognizing your child's talents, interests, and dreams. Support them in exploring paths that match their passions, like further education, work, or community involvement. Help your child imagine a future full of opportunities.

- ***Setting Realistic Goals:*** Collaborate with your child to set attainable goals. Break big goals into smaller steps, and celebrate each achievement. Goals should be meaningful to your child and reflect their unique abilities.

- ***Fostering Independence:*** Help your child become more independent by letting them practice life skills and make decisions. Support their autonomy while guiding them. Encouraging independence helps your child face adulthood with confidence.

Resources for Continued Support and Growth

Accessing ongoing support and resources is essential for your child's continued growth and development. Here are some valuable resources to consider:

- ***Support Groups and Networks:*** Join support groups and online communities for parents of autistic individuals. These offer a chance to share experiences and advice.

- ***Professional Services:*** Seek out professional services and specialists who can provide tailored support and guidance for your child's specific needs. This may include speech therapists, occupational therapists, behavioral therapists, or educational consultants who can offer personalized interventions and strategies.

- ***Transition Programs and Services:*** Investigate transition programs and services offered by your child's school, community organizations, or government agencies. These programs often provide support in areas such as vocational training, independent living skills, and job placement, helping your child transition smoothly into adulthood.

As you look to the future, remember you're not alone. By using resources, promoting independence, and supporting your child's interests, you set the stage for a future full of growth and potential. Let's move forward with hope, resilience, and a commitment to our children's success.

Conclusion

As we come to the end of this transformative journey, it's a moment to pause, reflect, and embrace the emotions that have accompanied us every step of the way. From the initial diagnosis to the countless milestones and challenges faced, our journey as parents of autistic teens has been a testament to resilience, love, and unwavering determination.

Reflecting on the Journey

As I look back on my own journey, I am reminded of the countless highs and lows, the moments of triumph and uncertainty that have shaped our path. I remember the fear and confusion that accompanied the initial diagnosis, the sleepless nights filled with worry and doubt about what the future held for my child. But I also recall the moments of sheer joy and pride as I witnessed my child's resilience, perseverance, and unique gifts shining through.

Final Thoughts and Encouragement

To all the parents walking this journey alongside me, I want you to know that you are not alone. I have felt the weight of your worries, the ache of your heartaches, and the overwhelming love that propels you forward, even in the darkest of times. I understand the fear of the unknown, the frustration of navigating systems that don't always understand or support our children's needs, and the bittersweet beauty of celebrating every small victory along the way.

But despite the challenges, I want to remind you of the incredible strength and resilience that resides within each of us. We are warriors, advocates, and champions for our children, and we will stop at nothing to ensure that they are seen, heard, and valued for who they are. Let us continue to lean on each other for support, to share our stories, our struggles, and our triumphs, knowing that together, we are stronger.

As we embark on the next chapter of our journey, let us carry with us the lessons learned, the bonds forged, and the hope that continues to guide us forward. Our children may face obstacles, setbacks, and hurdles along the way, but with our unwavering love, support, and belief in their potential, there is no limit to what they can achieve.

So, to every parent, caregiver, and advocate, I leave you with this: hold onto hope, cherish every moment, and never underestimate the power of love to light the way. Our journey may be challenging, but it is also filled with beauty, resilience, and boundless possibility. Together, let us continue to walk this path with courage, grace, and a fierce determination to create a world where all our children can thrive.